Healthy Gut Meal Plan

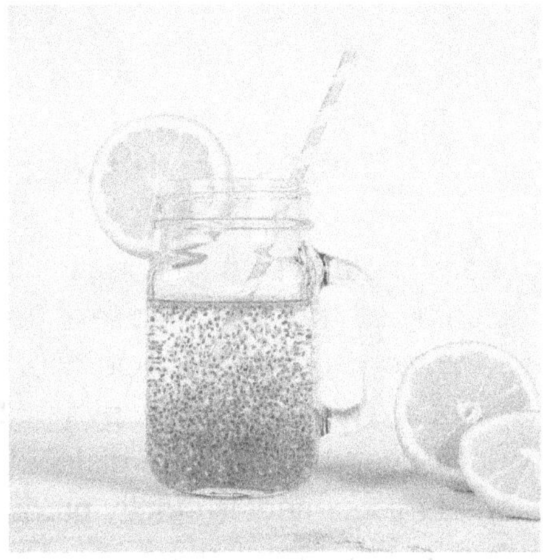

Gut Health and Digestive Health
Diets, Recipes and Meal Plan

ISAAC HENDRICKS

Table of Contents

INTRODUCTION

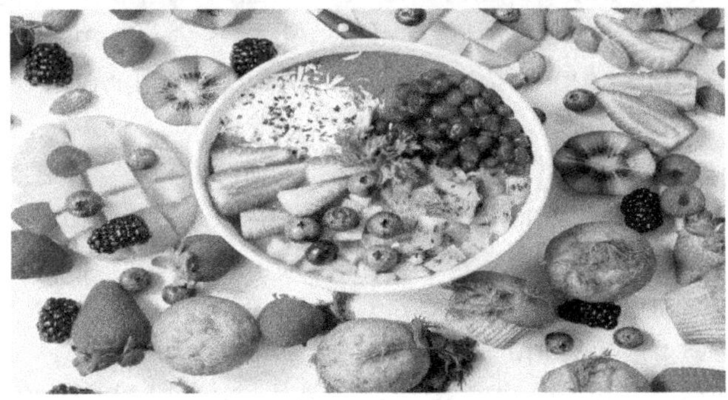

Once upon a time, in a world where people were becoming increasingly health-conscious, there was a woman named Mary. Mary had always struggled with digestive issues, and no matter what she ate, she seemed to have bloating, gas, and discomfort. She knew that she needed to make a change, and that's when she discovered the concept of a healthy gut meal plan.

A healthy gut meal plan is a dietary approach that focuses on promoting a healthy balance of bacteria in the gut. It involves eating foods that are rich in fibre, probiotics, and prebiotics, while avoiding foods that can cause inflammation and discomfort. Mary was intrigued by this concept, and she decided to give it a try.

At first, Mary found the meal plan challenging. She was used to eating processed foods and fast food, and she wasn't sure how to incorporate all of the new foods into her diet. But she was determined to make a change, and she started small. She began by adding more fruits and vegetables to her meals, and she found that she enjoyed the new flavours and textures.

As Mary continued to follow the meal plan, she noticed a significant improvement in her digestion. She no longer experienced bloating or discomfort after meals, and she felt more energised throughout the day. She also noticed that she was sleeping better and that her moods were more stable.

Mary's newfound success inspired her to share her story with others. She started a blog and a social media campaign, encouraging people to try the healthy gut meal plan for themselves. She also worked with a nutritionist to develop a meal plan that was tailored to her specific needs and preferences.

Through her blog and social media, Mary was able to connect with people from all over the world who were struggling with digestive issues. She shared recipes, tips, and advice, and she provided a supportive community for people to connect with.

Mary's story is a testament to the power of a healthy gut meal plan. It's not just about improving digestion, but also about promoting overall health and wellbeing. By making small changes to our diets, we can have a big impact on our bodies and our lives.

If you're interested in learning more about the healthy gut meal plan, I encourage you to check out Mary's blog and social media channels. She's a true inspiration, and her story is a reminder that we all have the power to take control of our health and wellbeing. Let's follow in Mary's footsteps and make a positive change in our lives, one meal at a time.

What is a Healthy Gut Meal Plan?

A healthy gut meal plan is a dietary approach focused on promoting optimal gut health by incorporating foods that nourish and support the gut microbiome. It involves consuming a balanced diet rich in probiotic and prebiotic foods, fiber, and essential nutrients to maintain a thriving gut ecosystem.

Why is a Healthy Gut Important?

Having a healthy gut is crucial as it plays a pivotal role in our overall well-being. A healthy gut contributes to better digestion, absorption of nutrients, improved immune function, disease prevention, and even mental health.

What Effect Does a Healthy Gut Have on Our Overall Health?

A healthy gut has a significant impact on various aspects of our health. It influences nutrient absorption, reducing the risk of nutritional deficiencies. Moreover, a healthy gut aids in the elimination of waste and toxins, enhancing overall detoxification and promoting a stronger immune system. Mental health is also closely linked to gut health, as the gut produces neurotransmitters that affect mood and cognition.

CHAPTER ONE

Understanding the Gut Microbiome

The human body is home to trillions of bacteria, which are referred to collectively as the microbiome. While the majority of these microbes reside in the gut, their role in maintaining overall health and wellbeing has only recently gained attention in the scientific community. In this article, we will delve into the intricacies of the gut microbiome, exploring its composition, functions, and implications for human health.

The gut microbiome is a complex ecosystem consisting of bacteria, viruses, fungi, and archaea. These microbes interact with each other and the host in various ways, forming a delicate balance that is essential for optimal health. The composition of the gut microbiome is influenced by several factors, including genetics, diet, environment, and antibiotic use.

One of the most significant findings in gut microbiome research is the role of bacteria in the production of essential nutrients. For instance, certain strains of bacteria are capable of synthesising vitamins K and B12, which are crucial for bone health and red blood cell formation, respectively. Moreover, these bacteria help to break down complex carbohydrates that the human body cannot digest, thereby contributing to energy production.

The gut microbiota is also important for the immune system. The gut is the largest immune organ in the body, and the microbiome helps to train the immune system to distinguish between foreign invaders and harmless microbes. This process, known as immune tolerance, is essential for preventing autoimmune diseases and allergies.

However, an imbalance in the gut microbiome, known as dysbiosis, has been linked to several health issues, including inflammatory bowel disease, obesity, and depression. Dysbiosis can result from a variety of factors, including antibiotic use, diet, and stress. For instance, a diet high in processed foods and sugar can lead to an overgrowth of pathogenic bacteria, which can exacerbate inflammation and contribute to chronic diseases.

The potential therapeutic applications of gut microbiome research are vast. One promising area of research is the use of probiotics, which are live bacteria that are beneficial to health, to restore balance to the gut microbiome. Probiotics have been shown to alleviate symptoms of various gastrointestinal disorders, such as irritable bowel syndrome and antibiotic-associated diarrhoea.

Another area of research is the use of faecal transplants, which involve transferring faecal matter from a healthy donor to a patient with gut dysbiosis. Faecal transplants have shown promising results in the treatment of recurrent Clostridium difficile infections, a severe and often life-threatening condition.

In conclusion, the gut microbiome is a complex and dynamic ecosystem that plays a crucial role in human health. Its composition, functions, and implications for human health are still being unravelled, and further research is needed to fully understand its potential therapeutic applications. However, the current evidence suggests that a healthy gut microbiome is essential for optimal health and wellbeing, and strategies to promote a balanced microbiome, such as a healthy diet and probiotic use, may have significant benefits for overall health.

The Role of Microorganisms in Our Gut

Trillions of microorganisms, including bacteria, viruses, fungus, and other microbes, live in our gut microbiome. These microorganisms play a vital role in maintaining gut health by aiding digestion, producing essential nutrients, and regulating immune function.

Factors Affecting the Gut Microbiota

Several factors can impact the

composition and diversity of our gut microbiota, such as diet, lifestyle, stress, medication use, and environmental factors. Understanding these influences can help us make informed choices to support a healthy gut.

The Connection Between Gut Health and Disease

Emerging research suggests that an imbalance in the gut microbiota, known as dysbiosis, may contribute to various health conditions, including obesity, diabetes, inflammatory bowel disease, and even mental health disorders. Maintaining a healthy gut through a well-designed meal plan can help prevent and manage these conditions.

CHAPTER TWO

Principles of a Healthy Gut Meal Plan

A healthy gut is vital for general health since it is involved in digestion, nutrition absorption, and immunological function. A gut-friendly meal plan can help promote a healthy gut by incorporating foods that are rich in fibre, probiotics, and prebiotics. Here are some principles to consider when creating a healthy gut meal plan:

1. Increase Fibre Intake

Fibre is essential for gut health as it promotes the growth of beneficial bacteria, prevents constipation, and reduces the risk of colon cancer. Aim to consume at least 25-30 grams of fibre per day from sources such as whole grains, fruits, vegetables, and legumes.

2. Incorporate Probiotics

Probiotics are live bacteria and yeasts that promote gut health by replenishing the good bacteria in the gut. Foods such as yoghurt, kefir, sauerkraut, kimchi, and miso are rich in probiotics.

3. Consume Prebiotics

Prebiotics are fibre-rich foods that feed the good bacteria in the gut, promoting their growth. Foods such as onions, garlic, asparagus, artichokes, and oats are rich in prebiotics.

4. Limit Processed Foods
Processed foods often contain additives, preservatives, and artificial sweeteners that can disrupt gut health. Reduce your intake of processed foods and replace them with full, unprocessed meals.

5. Manage Stress
Chronic stress can negatively impact gut health, leading to inflammation and digestive issues. Incorporate stress-reducing activities such as meditation, yoga, or deep breathing exercises into your daily routine.

6. Stay Hydrated
Drinking enough water is essential for gut health as it helps prevent constipation and promotes regular bowel movements. Drink at least eight glasses of water each day.

7. Limit Sugar and Artificial Sweeteners
Sugar and artificial sweeteners can negatively impact gut health by feeding the bad bacteria in the gut, leading to inflammation and digestive issues. Limit your intake of sugar and artificial sweeteners and opt for natural sweeteners such as honey, maple syrup, or stevia instead.

8. Practise Mindful Eating

Mindful eating involves paying attention to your food, savouring each bite, and eating slowly. This can help promote gut health by allowing your body to fully digest and absorb the nutrients from your food.

By incorporating these principles into your meal plan, you can promote a healthy gut and improve overall well-being. Remember to always consult with a healthcare professional or a registered dietitian for personalised advice based on your specific needs.

Balancing Macronutrients

A healthy gut meal plan emphasises a balanced intake of macronutrients - carbohydrates, proteins, and fats. Each nutrient plays a unique role in gut health, and finding the right balance promotes a thriving gut ecosystem.

Incorporating Fiber-Rich Foods

Dietary fiber is a crucial component of a healthy gut meal plan. It functions as a prebiotic, feeding healthy intestinal microorganisms. Including a variety of fiber-rich foods helps support regular bowel movements, lowers inflammation, and reduces the risk of chronic disease.

Introducing Fermented Foods

Fermented foods are key to promoting a healthy gut due to their high content of beneficial bacteria. Incorporating fermented foods into your meal plan, such as yogurt, sauerkraut, and kefir, increases the diversity of gut microbes, aiding digestion and overall gut health.

Promoting Digestive Enzyme Production

Optimising digestion is essential for maintaining a healthy gut. Choosing foods that promote the production of digestive enzymes, such as pineapple and papaya, can improve nutrient absorption and reduce digestive discomfort.

CHAPTER THREE

Foods to Include in a Healthy Gut Meal Plan

A healthy gut is essential for overall well-being as it houses trillions of beneficial bacteria that aid in digestion, boost immunity, and even impact mood and cognitive function. A diet rich in fibre, probiotics, and prebiotics can promote a healthy gut microbiome. Here are some foods to include in a healthy gut meal plan:

1. Fruits and Vegetables

Fruits and vegetables are rich in fibre, which promotes the growth of beneficial bacteria in the gut. Some great options include apples, berries, leafy greens, broccoli, and artichokes.

2. Whole Grains

Whole grains like oats, quinoa, and brown rice are high in fibre and prebiotics, which feed the beneficial bacteria in the gut.

3. Lean Proteins

Lean proteins like chicken, fish, and legumes are easy to digest and provide the body with essential amino acids.

4. Fermented Foods

Fermented foods like yoghourt, kefir, kimchi, sauerkraut, and kombucha contain probiotics, which are beneficial bacteria that promote a healthy gut microbiome.

5. Nuts and Seeds
Nuts and seeds like chia seeds, flaxseeds, and almonds are rich in fibre and healthy fats, which promote a healthy gut.

6. Herbal Teas
Herbal teas like ginger, peppermint, and chamomile can soothe the digestive system and promote a healthy gut.

7. Water
Staying hydrated is essential for a healthy gut as it helps to prevent constipation and promotes regular bowel movements.

By incorporating these foods into your diet, you can promote a healthy gut microbiome and improve overall health and well-being.

Probiotic Foods

Including probiotic-rich foods in your meal plan introduces beneficial bacteria into your gut, enhancing its health and function. Yoghurt, kefir, sauerkraut, kimchi, and kombucha are excellent sources of probiotics that can be easily incorporated into your daily meals.

Prebiotic Foods

Prebiotics are nondigestible fibers that serve as a source of nutrition for healthy gut flora. Garlic, onions, leeks, asparagus, and bananas are great examples of prebiotic foods that can be included in your healthy gut meal plan to support a flourishing gut microbiome.

Fibre-Rich Foods

Consuming a wide variety of fibre-rich foods, such as whole grains, legumes, fruits, and vegetables, provides numerous benefits for your gut. These meals enhance intestinal regularity, feed beneficial gut bacteria, and aid with weight management.

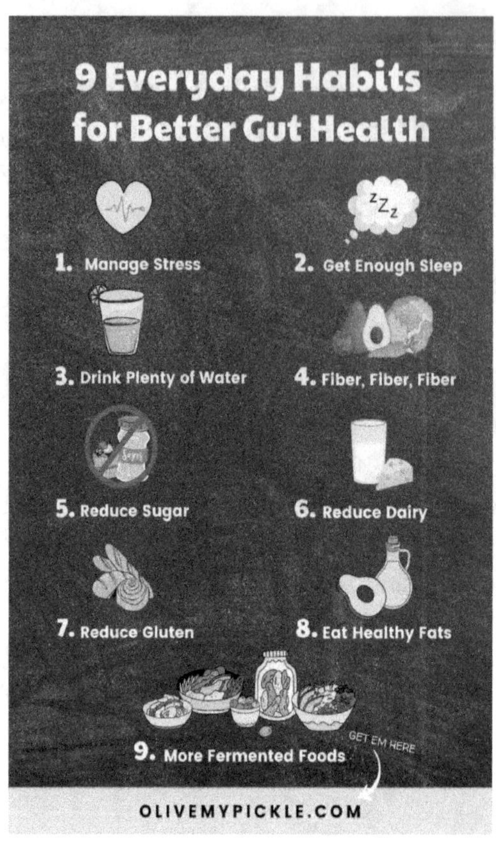

9 Everyday Habits
for Better Gut Health
1. Manage Stress
2. Get Enough Sleep
3. Drink Plenty of Water
4. Fiber, Fiber, Fiber
5. Reduce Sugar
6. Reduce Dairy
7. Reduce Gluten
8. Eat Healthy Fats
9. More Fermented Foods
GET EM HERE
OLIVEMYPICKLE.COM

CHAPTER FOUR

Foods to Avoid for a Healthy Gut

Maintaining a healthy gut is crucial for overall well-being as the gut is home to trillions of bacteria that play a vital role in digestion, nutrient absorption, and immune system function. While there are many foods that promote a healthy gut, there are also certain foods that should be avoided to prevent gut issues. For a healthy gut, avoid the following foods:

Processed and packaged foods

Processed and packaged foods often contain preservatives, additives, and artificial sweeteners that can disrupt the gut microbiome. These chemicals can cause inflammation, bloating, and diarrhoea.

Sugary and high-fat foods

Consuming too much sugar and fat can lead to an overgrowth of bad bacteria in the gut, causing inflammation and digestive issues.

Alcohol

Alcohol can irritate the gut lining, leading to inflammation and leaky gut syndrome. It can also

disrupt the gut microbiome, leading to an
overgrowth of bad bacteria.

Caffeine

Caffeine can stimulate the production of stomach
acid, leading to heartburn, acid reflux, and
indigestion.

Spicy foods

Spicy foods can irritate the gut lining, causing
inflammation and digestive issues.

Carbonated drinks

Carbonated drinks can cause bloating and gas,
leading to discomfort and digestive issues.

Gluten

For individuals with celiac disease or gluten
sensitivity, consuming gluten can lead to gut
inflammation, diarrhoea, and other digestive issues.

Dairy

For individuals with lactose intolerance, consuming
dairy can lead to bloating, gas, and diarrhoea.

Processed Foods and Refined Sugars

Processed foods and refined sugars can disrupt the
balance of gut bacteria, leading to inflammation and

dysbiosis. Avoiding processed snacks, sodas, and excessively sweetened foods is essential for preserving gut health.

Artificial Sweeteners

Artificial sweeteners, often found in diet soda, low-calorie foods, and sugar-free products, can negatively impact the gut microbiome. They may alter gut bacteria composition and affect overall gut health.

Trans Fats and Saturated Fats

Trans fats and saturated fats, commonly found in fried and processed foods, can promote inflammation and harm beneficial gut bacteria. Limiting the consumption of these unhealthy fats helps maintain gut health and reduces the risk of inflammation-related diseases.

Excessive Caffeine and Alcohol

While moderate consumption of caffeine and alcohol is generally acceptable, excessive intake can negatively affect the gut microbiome. Both caffeine and alcohol can disrupt the delicate balance of gut bacteria and contribute to gut inflammation.

By avoiding these foods, individuals can promote a healthy gut and prevent gut issues. Instead, they should focus on consuming a diet rich in fibre,

probiotics, and prebiotics to promote a healthy gut
microbiome. Some examples of gut-friendly foods
include leafy greens, berries, whole grains,
fermented foods like yoghourt and kefir, and
healthy fats like avocado and nuts.

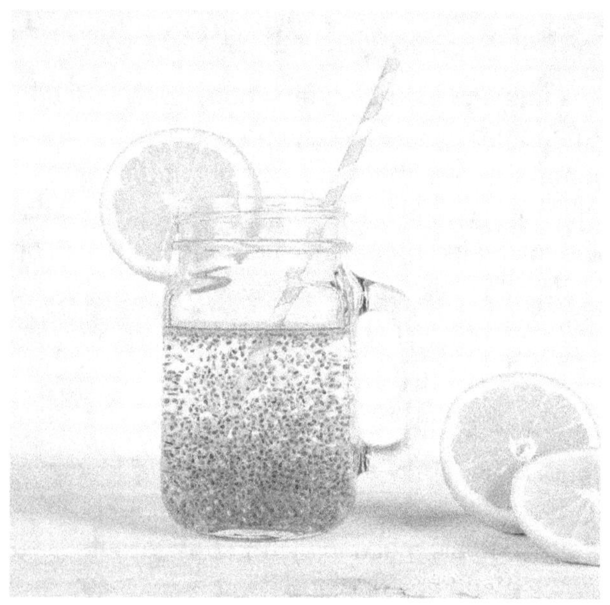

CHAPTER FIVE

Meal Planning Strategies for a Healthy Gut

Meal planning is a crucial aspect of maintaining a healthy gut. The gut is home to trillions of bacteria, collectively known as the gut microbiome, which play a significant role in our overall health and wellbeing. Proper digestion, nutritional absorption, and immunological function are all dependent on a healthy gut microbiota. Here are some meal planning strategies to promote a healthy gut:

Include fibre-rich foods

Fibre is essential for promoting healthy gut bacteria. It works as a prebiotic, feeding the good bacteria in the gut. Some high-fibre foods include fruits like apples, berries, and pears, vegetables like broccoli, kale, and artichokes, and whole grains like oats and quinoa.

Add probiotics

Probiotics are live bacteria and yeasts that are beneficial for gut health. They can be found in fermented foods like yoghourt, kefir, kimchi, and sauerkraut. Adding probiotics to your meal plan can help replenish the gut microbiome and promote a healthy balance of bacteria.

Limit processed foods

Processed foods often contain added sugars, preservatives, and artificial sweeteners that can negatively impact gut health. They can disrupt the gut microbiome and lead to inflammation and digestive issues. Instead, eat as many complete, unadulterated meals as possible.

Incorporate healthy fats

Healthy fats, such as those found in avocados, nuts, and olive oil, can promote a healthy gut microbiome. They can also help absorb fat-soluble vitamins and minerals.

Practise mindful eating

Mindful eating involves paying attention to your food, savouring each bite, and eating slowly. This can help promote healthy digestion and prevent overeating, which can lead to discomfort and digestive issues.

Stay hydrated

Drinking enough water is crucial for maintaining a healthy gut. Water helps move food through the digestive system and prevent constipation. Aim for eight glasses of water per day.

Consider working with a registered dietitian

If you have digestive issues or want to optimise your gut health, working with a registered dietitian can be helpful. They can provide personalised meal planning advice based on your unique needs and goals.

Building Balanced Meals

Designing well-balanced meals ensures you receive an adequate intake of essential nutrients while supporting gut health. Incorporating lean proteins, whole grains, healthy fats, and a variety of fruits and vegetables in each meal is essential.

Creating Variety in Your Diet

Introducing a wide range of foods in your meal plan promotes gut microbiota diversity. Experiment with various vegetables, fruits, whole grains, and proteins to provide a diverse array of nutrients to your gut bacteria.

Modifying Recipes for Gut Health

By making simple modifications to your favourite recipes, you can transform them into gut-friendly meals. Swap refined grains with whole grains, use healthy fats, and add fermented or prebiotic-rich ingredients to boost gut health.

Smart Snacking Tips

Snacking can be a part of a healthy gut meal plan if done wisely. Choose nutritious options such as fresh fruits, nuts, seeds, or yoghurt, and pay attention to portion sizes. Avoid highly processed snacks and opt for whole food options instead.

By incorporating these meal planning strategies into your routine, you can promote a healthy gut microbiome and overall gut health. Remember to always consult with a healthcare professional if you have any concerns or questions regarding your gut health.

CHAPTER SIX

Benefits and Challenges of a Healthy Gut Meal Plan

A healthy gut meal plan refers to a dietary approach that focuses on promoting the growth of beneficial bacteria in the gut, improving digestion, and reducing inflammation. This meal plan has gained popularity in recent years due to its numerous health benefits, but it also presents some challenges. In this article, we will explore the benefits and challenges of a healthy gut meal plan.

Benefits of a Healthy Gut Meal Plan

1. Improved Digestion:
A healthy gut meal plan is rich in fibre, which helps to promote regular bowel movements and prevent constipation. Fibre also feeds the beneficial bacteria in the gut, which in turn helps to improve digestion and reduce bloating and gas.

2. Reduced Inflammation:
The gut is home to a diverse range of bacteria, some of which can contribute to inflammation in the body. A healthy gut meal plan includes foods that are anti-inflammatory, such as leafy greens,

berries, and fatty fish, which can help to reduce inflammation and improve overall health.

3. Improved Mental Health:
The gut and the brain are closely connected, and a healthy gut meal plan has been shown to improve mental health. For example, foods rich in probiotics, such as yoghourt and kefir, can help to reduce symptoms of anxiety and depression.

4. Weight Management:
A healthy gut meal plan can also help with weight management. Foods that are high in fibre, such as fruits, vegetables, and whole grains, can help to keep you feeling full for longer, which can prevent overeating and promote weight loss.

Challenges of a Healthy Gut Meal Plan

1. Limited Food Choices:
A healthy gut meal plan can be restrictive, as it may exclude certain foods that are high in sugar, processed ingredients, and unhealthy fats. This can make it challenging to find new and interesting meal ideas, and it may require some creativity in the kitchen.

2. Cost:
Some of the foods that are recommended in a healthy gut meal plan, such as organic produce and grass-fed meat, can be expensive. This can make it

challenging for people with limited budgets to follow this meal plan.

3. Time Constraints:
Preparing healthy meals can be time-consuming, especially if you are trying to incorporate a variety of foods into your diet. This can be difficult for folks who have busy schedules or poor cooking skills.

4. Adjustment Period:
Changing your diet can be challenging, and it may take some time for your body to adjust to a healthy gut meal plan. During this adjustment period, you may experience some digestive discomfort, such as bloating or gas, as your body adjusts to the new foods.

In conclusion, a healthy gut meal plan has numerous health benefits, but it also presents some challenges. By being aware of these challenges and finding ways to overcome them, such as meal planning, budgeting, and seeking out new recipes, you can enjoy the benefits of a healthy gut meal plan while still enjoying a variety of delicious and nutritious foods.

Improved Digestion and Nutrient Absorption

A healthy gut meal plan supports proper digestion and optimal absorption of nutrients, leading to improved gut health and overall well-being.

Enhanced digestion can reduce bloating, gas, and discomfort.

Enhanced Immune System

A healthy gut strengthens the immune system, as approximately 70% of our immune cells are located in the gut. A well-nourished gut microbiota can help prevent infections, allergies, and other immune system-related disorders.

Potential Weight Management

Maintaining a healthy gut through a balanced meal plan may support weight management efforts. Gut bacteria influence our metabolism, hunger signals, and fat storage, making a healthy gut pivotal for maintaining a healthy weight.

Overcoming Common Hurdles

Transitioning to a healthy gut meal plan may present challenges, such as taste preferences, limited time for meal preparation, and social pressures. Finding creative ways to adapt recipes and seeking support from others can help overcome these hurdles.

Adjusting to a New Way of Eating

Adjusting to a new way of eating takes time and patience. Gradual changes, seeking recipe inspiration, and understanding the long-term

benefits of a healthy gut meal plan can help ease
the transition and ensure long-term success.

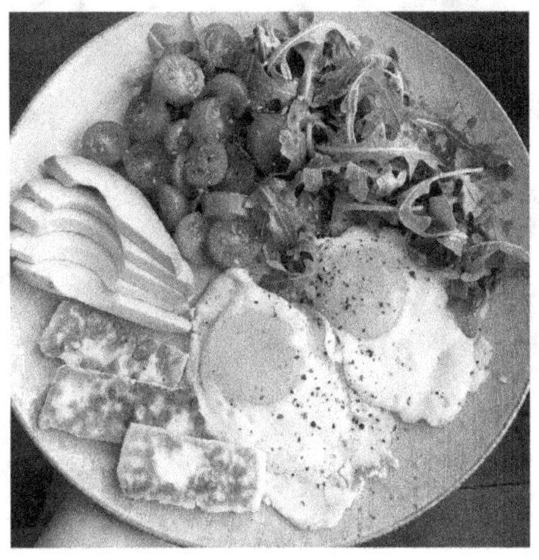

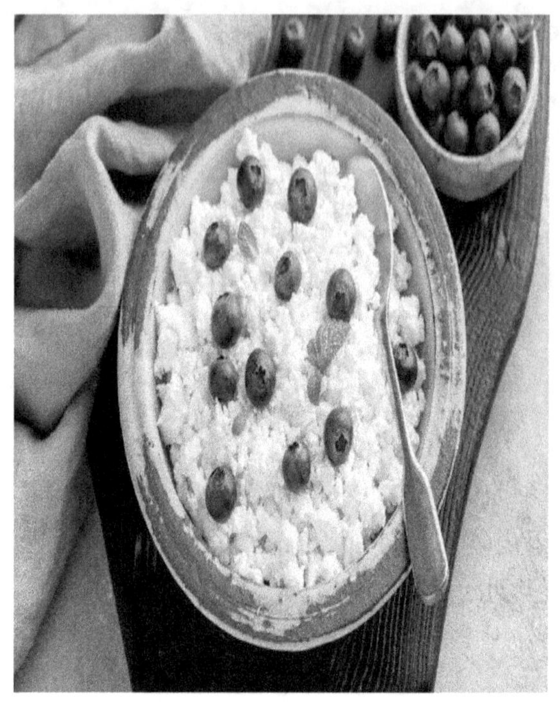

CHAPTER SEVEN

FAQs on Gut Health and Meal Planning

1. What is gut health?

Gut health refers to the overall well-being of the digestive system, which includes the stomach, intestines, and colon. A healthy gut is essential for proper digestion, nutrient absorption, and the prevention of diseases.

2. How can I improve my gut health?

There are various things you may do to improve your gut health, including:

- Consuming a fibre-rich, probiotic- and prebiotic-rich diet
- Staying hydrated
- Managing stress
- Getting enough sleep
- Exercising regularly
- Limiting processed foods and sugar intake
- Avoiding smoking and excessive alcohol consumption

3. What foods are good for gut health?

Foods that are good for gut health include:

- Fruits and vegetables, especially those high in fibre such as berries, leafy greens, and cruciferous vegetables
- Oatmeal, quinoa, and brown rice are examples of whole grains.
- Fermented foods such as yoghourt, kefir, kimchi, and sauerkraut
- Nuts and seeds, especially chia seeds and flaxseeds
- Chicken, fish, and lentils are good sources of lean protein.

4. What foods should I avoid for gut health?

Foods that should be avoided or limited for gut health include:

- Sugary and fattening processed foods and snacks
- Carbonated drinks and sugary beverages
- Fried foods and fast food
- Excessive alcohol consumption
- Spicy foods for those with sensitive stomachs

5. How can I make a meal plan for gut health?

Meal planning for gut health involves:

- Choosing whole, nutrient-dense foods
- Incorporating a variety of fibre-rich foods

- Including fermented foods for probiotics
- Limiting processed foods and sugary beverages
- Planning for balanced meals with protein, fibre, and healthy fats
- Planning meals ahead of time to avoid making poor choices at the last minute.

6. How can I manage gut health concerns such as bloating and constipation?

To manage gut health concerns such as bloating and constipation, consider:

- Increasing fibre intake gradually to avoid bloating
- Consuming enough of water to avoid constipation
- Exercising regularly to promote bowel movements
- Stress management with relaxation techniques or exercise
- Consulting a healthcare provider for persistent symptoms

7. What are some gut health supplements I can consider?

Some gut health supplements to consider include:

- Probiotics to promote a healthy gut bacteria balance
- Digestive enzymes to aid in digestion
- Magnesium citrate for constipation relief
- Slippery elm to soothe an irritated gut

- Marshmallow root to reduce inflammation

8. How can I ensure I am getting enough nutrients with a gut health-focused diet?

To ensure you are getting enough nutrients with a gut health-focused diet, consider:

- Eating a variety of whole, nutrient-dense foods
- Incorporating magnesium, iron, and vitamin D-rich meals
- Consulting a healthcare provider or a registered dietitian for personalized nutritional guidance
- Taking a multivitamin supplement if necessary

9. How can I make gut health-focused meals more flavorful?

To make gut health-focused meals more flavorful, consider:

- Using herbs and spices such as turmeric, ginger, and cinnamon
- Experimenting with different cooking methods such as grilling, roasting, or steaming
- Adding healthy fats such as olive oil, avocado, or nuts for flavour and nutrition
- Trying new recipes and cuisines to keep meals interesting

10. How can I maintain gut health while eating out or travelling?

To maintain gut health while eating out or travelling, consider:

- Choosing restaurants that offer healthy, whole food options
- Avoiding processed and sugary foods
- Packing healthy snacks and meals for travel
- Drinking plenty of water to stay hydrated
- Choosing foods that are familiar and easy to digest
- Washing your hands frequently and refraining from touching your face
- Consulting a healthcare provider for travel-related health concerns.

11. Can a Healthy Gut Meal Plan Help with Digestive Disorders?

A healthy gut meal plan can indeed help manage digestive disorders such as irritable bowel syndrome (IBS) or inflammatory bowel disease (IBD). By focusing on gut-friendly foods and avoiding triggers, symptoms can be reduced, and gut health can be improved.

12. Is it Necessary to Take Probiotic Supplements if Following a Healthy Gut Diet?

While probiotic supplements can be beneficial, it is not always necessary to take them if you are following a healthy gut meal plan. A well-balanced diet rich in probiotic and prebiotic foods can provide sufficient beneficial bacteria to support gut health.

13. Can a Healthy Gut Meal Plan Aid in Weight Loss?

A healthy gut meal plan, combined with regular physical activity, can support weight loss efforts. The diverse gut microbiota that results from a healthy gut diet enhances metabolism, digestion, and absorption of nutrients, favoring weight management.

14. How Long Does it Take to Notice Changes in Gut Health?

The time it takes to notice changes in gut health varies for each individual. Generally, noticeable improvements may occur within a few weeks to a few months, depending on the current state of your gut and adherence to a healthy gut meal plan.

CONCLUSION

Final Thoughts and Tips for Maintaining a Healthy Gut Meal Plan

Final Thoughts

Maintaining a healthy gut is essential for overall well-being, and a meal plan focused on gut health can significantly improve digestion, reduce inflammation, and boost immunity. Here are some final thoughts and tips for sticking to a gut-healthy meal plan:

1. Be consistent:
Consistency is key when it comes to maintaining a healthy gut. Try to eat gut-friendly foods regularly to see the best results.

2. Pay attention to your body:
Pay attention to how your body reacts to various foods. Some people may have sensitivities to certain foods, such as gluten or dairy, that can negatively impact gut health.

3. Incorporate variety:

Eating a variety of gut-friendly foods can help ensure that you're getting all the necessary nutrients for optimal gut health.

4. Manage stress:

Chronic stress can negatively impact gut health, so finding ways to manage stress, such as meditation or yoga, can be beneficial.

5. Stay hydrated:

Drinking plenty of water throughout the day can help promote healthy digestion and prevent constipation.

6. Consult a healthcare professional:

If you have ongoing gut issues, it may be helpful to consult a healthcare professional, such as a registered dietitian or gastroenterologist, for personalized advice and guidance.

Tips for Maintaining a Healthy Gut Meal Plan

1. Incorporate gut-friendly foods:

Some gut-friendly foods to include in your meal plan are probiotic-rich foods like yogurt, kefir, and kimchi, prebiotic-rich foods like onions, garlic, and asparagus, and fiber-rich foods like whole grains, fruits, and vegetables.

2. Limit processed foods:

Processed foods often contain added sugars, preservatives, and artificial ingredients that can negatively impact gut health.

3. Choose lean protein sources:
Lean protein sources like chicken, fish, and legumes can help promote healthy digestion and prevent constipation.

4. Cook foods properly:
Cooking foods properly, such as thoroughly cooking meats and vegetables, can help prevent foodborne illnesses and promote healthy digestion.

5. Practice portion control:
Eating too much of any food, even gut-friendly foods, can lead to discomfort and digestive issues.

6. Plan ahead:
Planning meals ahead of time can help ensure that you're making healthy choices and sticking to your gut-healthy meal plan.

In conclusion, maintaining a healthy gut is crucial for overall well-being, and a meal plan focused on gut health can significantly improve digestion, reduce inflammation, and boost immunity. By following these tips and staying consistent, you can promote healthy gut function and enjoy the many benefits of a gut-healthy diet.
A healthy gut meal plan is a powerful tool for supporting gut health and overall well-being. By

incorporating probiotic and prebiotic foods, fibre-rich foods, and following mindful meal planning strategies, you can establish a foundation for long-term gut health. Remember to listen to your body, adapt your plan accordingly, and seek professional guidance if needed.

www.ingramcontent.com/pod-product-compliance
Lightning Source LLC
Chambersburg PA
CBHW071008260726
48661CB00007B/2860